Superfoods that Kickstart Your Weight Loss

BY LINDSEY P

Learn How to Use 60 Superfoods to Boost Weight Loss, Immunity and to Live a Healthier Lifestyle

Table of Contents

Introduction

I want to thank you and congratulate you for purchasing the book, "Superfoods that Kick Start Your Weight Loss: Learn How to Use 30 Superfoods to Boost Weight Loss, Immunity and to Live a Healthier Lifestyle".

This book contains proven steps and strategies on how to know which foods to eat to speed up your weight loss and feel and look healthier too. Further, since superfoods cannot give you any benefits if you do not eat them, this book will also teach you various ideas on how to enjoy them.

Thanks again for purchasing this book, I hope you enjoy it!

Chapter 1 –Supermarket Staples

Though it is easy to think that superfoods are all exotic items from the jungles of a different continent, the truth is many of them can be found in your local supermarket. Here are the best supermarket superfoods:

1. Oats

When people start trying to lose weight, one problem they have is how to deal with the decreased amount of food without getting hungry. The answer is fiber. Fiber-rich foods are digested in the stomach at a slower rate compared to other foods which means that your stomach remains full for longer which, in turn, means that you *feel* full longer. This is why it is advisable to start the day with a fiber-rich cereal like oatmeal.

While fiber-rich cold cereals may seem like a great idea for those on the go, a hot breakfast can perk you up especially during the colder seasons. Instant oatmeal only takes a few minutes to cook in the microwave or if you heat water for your tea, add an extra cup to cook your oatmeal. Alternatively, you can cook up a batch of oatmeal at the beginning of the week and heat a bowl in the microwave every morning.

In addition to keeping you full for longer, the fiber in oatmeal, known as beta-glucan, is scientifically proven to help lower cholesterol levels. Studies have shown that cholesterol levels can drop up to 20% if a cup of oatmeal is consumed daily.

If that isn't enough for you, further studies show that oats contain the antioxidant avenanthramides which helps prevent cardiovascular disease. Beta-glucan has been shown to improve the immune system by making the body more effective in fighting bacteria. Lastly, even if you flavor your oatmeal with a lot of sugar, the fiber will prevent spikes in your blood sugar thus preventing type-II diabetes in the long run. This is not to say, however, that you should make your cereal extremely sweet.

Here are some ideas to flavor your oatmeal. If you make a batch of oatmeal at the beginning of the week to reheat in the mornings, make it unflavored so you can vary your sweeteners or flavorings depending on your mood:

To each bowl of oatmeal, add any of the following or a combination:

- A handful of berries

- Honey and Greek yoghurt

- Applesauce

If you become sick of oatmeal, here are other ideas to get your oat fix for the day:

- Add a cup of oatmeal to your favorite pancake batter recipe. Decrease the liquid by half a cup or depending on how watery your oatmeal is.

2. Apples

We've all heard the cliché about an apple a day, but most of us don't know why this is said. Besides the truth that eating more fruits and vegetables can make us healthier, eating more apples can help with weight loss by providing fiber which makes us feel full for longer. The fiber in apples is called pectin, and according to studies it can lower cholesterol levels too.

Apples are a great snack to ward off hunger pangs in between meals. A medium apple will contain about 90 calories and will make you feel more satisfied compared to 2 2-inch chocolate chip cookies which will also provide the same amount of calories. Ripe apples will give you your sweet fix.

In addition to fiber, apples also contain antioxidants called flavonoids which help prevent cancer in the long-run. They can also keep cholesterol levels at bay.

Munching on apples is a great way to enjoy this fruit, but if you're a little bored with this, you can do the following:

- Add slices of apple to your chicken or turkey sandwiches

- Sprinkle apple slices with cinnamon and a little honey

- Core an apple and fill the hole with a tablespoon of peanut butter

Stay away from apple pies, fritters and other sugary apple desserts. The sugar and calorie content will cancel out the benefits you get from the apples.

3. Sweet potatoes

While baked white potatoes can be good for you as long as you don't overload them with butter, cheese and other fattening toppings, swapping them for baked sweet potatoes will give you extras like more fiber, more vitamin A and C, more potassium and calcium, and extras like manganese and magnesium. You also get all these extras for fewer calories.

You can replace white potatoes for sweet potatoes in many recipes, and you can use mashed sweet potatoes as a sweetener for your baked goods, pancakes or waffles. This will give them a boost in nutritional value and lessen the calorie count from sugar.

However, take care when eating sweet potato desserts, fries or fritters. As with apple desserts, these food items may contain too much sugar and fat.

Here are some ideas for sweet potatoes:

- For a quick meal, you can microwave sweet potatoes. Wash them then dry thoroughly. Pierce them all over with a fork then lay on a microwave-safe dish. Cover with a damp paper towel. Microwave them on high for five minutes. Do this as often as necessary until they feel soft to the touch. (Be careful since they will be hot.) Add a dash of cinnamon, nutmeg, or brown sugar for a sweet meal, or add a tablespoon of cheese, diced tomatoes, or a drizzle of olive oil for a savory meal.

- Microwave several sweet potatoes and keep the rest in the fridge for a quick bite during lazy nights. You can also mash the sweet potato and add them to macaroni and cheese, your favorite pasta sauce or meatloaf recipes.

4. Hot Peppers

If you like hot foods, you're in luck. According to research, hot peppers can help you lose weight because of a wonderful compound called capsaicin. This compound can increase your metabolism by 3% even while you are at rest. If this does not seem like a lot, you should know too that capsaicin helps to curb your appetite by affecting the hormones which make you feel hungry.

There have been studies which suggest that capsaicin can prevent or lessen fatty deposits in the liver. Another study suggests that this compound helps the body digest carbohydrates and burn energy more efficiently. It may also increase energy levels.

Hot peppers also contain antioxidants like carotenoids and flavonoids which help to slow down aging and minimize the chances of getting cancer.

You can add hot peppers to sauces, stir-fry, stews or wherever you want. Depending on your preference, here are the various peppers from the hottest to the mildest:

- Ghost pepper

- Habanero

- Thai pepper

- Cayenne pepper

- Serrano pepper

- Jalapeno pepper

5. Herbs and spices

Enthusiastic cooks like to sprinkle their concoctions with herbs and spices to make them taste sophisticated and look special, but did you know that they can also suppress the appetite and increase metabolism? Here are the best choices and some ingenious ways to add more of them to your diet.

To suppress the appetite:

- Parsley – sprinkle on all savory dishes to add a fresh splash of green, make parsley pesto or chew on fresh sprigs to freshen the breath and clear the palate.

- Mint – chop and add to water for a refreshing drink especially during the summer, add to tea while steeping or chew fresh sprigs in between meals.

- Fennel – add to salads

To increase metabolism:

- Cinnamon – add to coffee, yoghurt, oatmeal

- Cardamom – add to coffee, desserts

- Ginger – grate and boil to make tea (Use ½ teaspoon to 1 cup of water and adjust to your taste), add to stir-fry

- Ginseng – use supplements or boil to make tea. (Follow the same method as for ginger.)

- Mustard – use to flavor mayonnaise, salad dressing, etc.

To lessen fat absorption:

- Turmeric – grate and boil to make tea. (Follow the same method as for ginger.)

- Black pepper – use more freshly cracked pepper on all you recipes

6. Nuts

Though nuts are fatty and calorific, they contain the good kind of unsaturated fats. If you are trying to lose weight, use nuts as treats or as a crunchy garnish on salads or cereals. This way you get the nutritional benefits without going overboard on the calories.

The best nuts you can eat are almonds and pistachios. Almonds are rich in vitamin E and can help lower cholesterol as well as help stabilize blood sugar levels. Meanwhile, pistachios are also rich in vitamin E and contain only 4 calories each which means you can splurge on them.

7. Milk

We are now advised to drink milk to prevent osteoporosis, but it contains more nutrients than just protein, calcium and vitamin D. Milk is also high in vitamin B2 and B12 and contains the minerals phosphorous, selenium and potassium. The one caveat with milk for those trying to lose weight is its fat content, but this is easily solved by choosing low-fat or non-fat milk.

Those who dislike the taste of milk can get its nutritional benefits by adding it to other food items like baked goods, pancakes and desserts. Here are some suggestions:

- Add an extra ¼ cup of non-fat dry milk to your pancake batter. This will make your pancakes creamier.

- Feel like a kid again by making the classic milk-cornstarch pudding and vary your flavorings depending on your mood. For those who have forgotten how make this dessert, here's the recipe:

Combine ¼ cup cornstarch with 3 cups of low-fat or skim milk and ¼ cup sugar or low-fat sweetener. Add 1 teaspoon of vanilla and your chosen flavorings, e.g. chocolate, cinnamon, almond, etc. Constantly stir over medium heat until thickened.

8. Salmon and other oily fish

While all kinds of fish are great when you wish to cut back on saturated fat, the oily kinds like salmon, tuna and mackerel provide omega-3 in the form of fish oil. It might seem contradictory to eat fatty food when you are trying to lose weight, but research suggests that omega-3 can assist in faster weight loss if it is combined with regular exercise because it encourages the body to use up fat stores for energy during exercise.

That said, remember that calories still matter when you are trying to lose weight. Try to balance calorific fatty fish with a low-calorie side like a green salad or whole grains. Also, avoid cooking methods which add calories like deep frying or cooking in butter. Avoid smothering the fish in cream or butter-based sauces as well.

Here are some ideas for salmon or other oily fish:

- Marinate fish fillets for 30 minutes in ponzu, a citrus flavored soy sauce, before grilling

- A new idea for canned tuna is to make tuna-potato cakes. Mix the tuna with mashed potatoes, season with salt, pepper and parsley and form into patties. Cook them on a lightly oiled pan until golden brown.

9. Berries

Berries are like small, nutritionally dense candies. If you have a sweet tooth, you're better off munching on a handful of berries than on candy. A cup of berries will have around 50 calories. That's a lot less than in a cup of candies. They are rich in vitamin C and provide some fiber too.

Since ripe berries are already sweet, try to avoid adding sugar to them since this will lessen their nutritional value. Here are some new ways to enjoy berries:

- Use crushed berries to replace the sugary jelly in peanut butter and jelly sandwiches

- Pulverize with yoghurt and freeze in popsicle molds

10. Beans

Beans are a great way to go meat-less during certain days. Meat, even if lean, contains saturated fat, and too much of this kind of fat can result in heart disease. A great way to lessen your saturated fat intake is to increase your vegetarian meals.

Beans are also a great diet staple since they are high in fiber and can make you feel full for longer. They can also help to regulate your blood sugar thus helping you avoid type-II diabetes in the long-run. They can help stretch a tight food budget or can add extra protein if meat is too expensive. But perhaps the best thing about them is they have fewer calories than meat. Try to eat a bean-based meal after splurging in high-calorie foods.

For beans to be a good source of protein, they should be combined with grains either in the same dish or in the same meal. This is because beans and grains by themselves do not contain all the essential amino acids the human body needs to make protein. They each have to provide the amino acids they lack.

In addition to protein and fiber, beans are rich in the B vitamins as well as in calcium.

Here are some ideas for adding more beans to your diet:

- Reduce or replace the meat in chili and add more kidney beans

- Mash cooked beans and add to chopped vegetables to make croquettes or veggie burgers

- Replace the tuna, egg or chicken in salads with mashed cooked white beans

11. Tofu

Another way to eat more beans is to eat tofu. If you don't like beans, tofu can be a way of incorporating more vegetarian meals to your lifestyle because you can easily make it taste whatever you want it to taste. Tofu can easily absorb flavors, either sweet or savory, and can take the form of various textures to simulate meat as much as possible.

For example, you can use tofu slices to replace meat cutlets or crumbled tofu to replace ground meat. You can use silken tofu to replace eggs in your cakes and to make a less calorific cake frosting.

Here is a recipe for tofu chocolate frosting:

1 square block of silken tofu (Make sure you get the silken kind and not the firm tofu)

1 teaspoon vanilla

1 cup semi-sweet chocolate chips

Combine the tofu and vanilla in a food processor. Melt the chocolate on a double boiler or in the microwave. Combine the chocolate with the tofu mixture and blend again until smooth.

12. Dark chocolate

Perhaps of all the superfoods, this is what most people would consider the best. Dark chocolate, if eaten in reasonable amounts, provide antioxidants which help prevent heart disease and cancer.

Choose chocolate products with the highest percentage of cocoa and with the least amount of sugar. The higher the percentage of cocoa, the more bitter it will taste. Generally, chocolate made with 70% cocoa will taste bitter to most people, so start with 50% cocoa and move up once you are used to the bitter taste.

When eating or cooking with dark chocolate, try to avoid mixing it with milk. Studies have shown that milk can prevent the absorption of antioxidants in dark chocolate. You can look up chocolate recipes using dark chocolate, or you can just eat it as is.

However, take note that too much of a good thing can be bad, and this is especially true of foods which taste good like dark chocolate. Use this as a treat instead of a meal.

Chapter 2 – The Exotics

While the above items can be easily found in most supermarkets, those listed here might be a little more difficult to find. Health food stores will sell these kinds of foods and you can also obtain them from the internet.

1. Quinoa

Native to the South American continent, this grain-like seed is high in protein, has concentrated amounts of antioxidants and provides heart-healthy monounsaturated fats.

Though some people like to think of it as a grain or cereal, technically speaking, since it isn't a member of the grass family like wheat or rice are, it is considered a pseudo-cereal. Regardless, quinoa is cooked and served in similar ways as most grains. You can serve it with lean meats for lunch and dinner, as a cereal for breakfast and as a nutritious addition to your baked goods, soups and stews. Quinoa can be bought as the whole seed and can come in white, black or red colors. Red and white quinoa have similar tastes while the black variety can taste a bit sweeter. You can also buy quinoa flakes which look and can be cooked like oatmeal. Quinoa flour can be added to your favorite baked goods recipes.

Regarding weight loss, quinoa is slightly more calorific than wheat or rice, but since it provides complete protein unlike grains, you can make it a part of a vegetarian meal which, on the whole, will contain fewer calories compared to a meal with an animal protein source.

Serve quinoa as you would most grains, or you can try the following:

- Lessen the meat in your stir-fry and add a cup of cooked quinoa

- Replace the ground meat in your chili recipe with quinoa

2. Goji berries

Also known as wolf berries, these small red berries are usually sold dried. They are native to China and the Chinese commonly use them in their medicinal soups and brews.

Goji berries have been proven to treat and prevent common lifestyle diseases like type-II diabetes and high blood pressure. They have also been proven to increase mental well-being. Perhaps if you are a stress eater, you are better off with goji berries than a bag of candies.

However, take note that they might interfere with certain drugs particularly blood thinners. It is best to check with your doctor if you are taking prescription medication before you try goji berries.

That said, if used non-medicinally, dried goji berries can be a great alternative to raisins and other dried fruit. They are slightly sweet and tart. You can also add a few to your tea pot while the tea is brewing. They will give a slight sweetness to the tea. You should consume the stewed berries to avoid wasting them.

Here are other ideas for goji berries:

- Use fresh berries if you can find them or rehydrate the dried ones in hot water and add to muffins, pancakes, waffles or other quick breads

- Combine goji berry with other red fruits to make a jam

- Mix with your favorite granola, cookie or brownie recipe

3. Wheat grass

Wheat grass supplement is now commonly found in juice bars and in health food stores as a concentrated source of nutrients. According to research, it contains high amounts of vitamin A, C, E, iron and calcium. It can lessen the complications of diabetes, lower high blood pressure, remove toxins from the liver and blood, cure infections and prevent cancer. It can also supposedly improve common ailments like the common cold, sore throat, fever, cough and joint pains.

If that sounds too good to be true, take note that the taste needs some getting used to. If you are a person who thinks green tea tastes too grassy, you will not like wheat grass. Fortunately, the common way of taking wheat grass is to mix it with juice.

With only 15 calories in one shot, you can easily add wheat grass to your morning glass of fruit juice. Take it every day for a week to see if gives you any benefits. Research says that a wheat grass shot is best consumed immediately after extraction so stay away from wheat grass powders.

4. Spirulina

Another grassy superfood is spirulina which is a blue-green algae that is dried and ground into powder or made into pills. Like wheat grass, it is a concentrated source of nutrients; but unlike wheat grass it contains protein, vitamin B complex, omega 3, 6 and 9, iron, calcium, and others.

If you have chosen to become vegetarian or vegan for the weight loss benefits, you can take spirulina supplements to boost your protein, iron and vitamin B12 intake.

Here are some great ways to add spirulina to your diet:

- Add spirulina powder to vegetable fritters

- Add a small amount of spirulina to your smoothies

- Sprinkle spirulina onto vegetable stir-fry

5. Acai

The acai berry is another superfood from South America. It is proven to be rich in antioxidants, even richer than the more common berries like strawberries and blueberries.

Unfortunately, acai has not yet been proven to be effective for weight loss; but since it is a nutritionally dense food, feel free to munch on them regularly. This way, you will not short-charge yourself on nutrition even if you maintain a reduced-calorie diet.

6. Camu Camu

Just like acai, camu camu is another wonder fruit from the same continent. It is reported to be very rich in vitamin C. One camu camu berry has 60 times more vitamin C than one orange. This is great news if you are prone to infections like the common cold or need to heal from wounds or skin ailments.

Camu camu tastes tart and citrusy. It is usually not consumed fresh since it can be very sour. You can buy camu camu powder, juice or capsules. Mix the powder or juice with other foods to tame down the taste.

7. Chia seeds

Most people think of a pet when they hear the word 'chia' but this word also refers to a superfood which is used to add protein, calcium and omega-3 to the diet. It can also help to stabilize blood sugar levels and lower cholesterol.

According to research, chia seeds can also help the body melt fat, especially the stubborn belly fat. They can also curb cravings by filling up the stomach much like other high-fiber foods do.

Unlike quinoa, chia is usually not eaten as is. You can add chia seeds to baked goods, sprinkled on salads or added to smoothies.

8. Edamame

Edamame is actually just boiled green soy beans served from the pod. In the previous chapter, we have discussed the benefits of eating tofu, but since soy beans are not commonly eaten fresh, most people are not familiar with this. Edamame will provide complete protein so you don't have to worry about combining the beans with grains as in most vegetarian meals.

As a snack, edamame contains fewer calories than nuts. You only consume about 120 calories for ½ cup, and it will give you 9 grams of fiber and 11 grams of protein. If you are the sort of person who pops peanuts in your mouth mindlessly, try this less calorific treat.

9. Star fruit

From South America, now we move to Asia. Star fruit is a star-shaped fruit which is high in vitamin C and antioxidants but low in calories. The unripe fruit can be very sour, but they sweeten when ripe. Due to their interesting shape, these fruits make a great garnish when sliced crosswise.

Add star fruit to your salads or add them to your smoothies for a refreshing tart taste. For only 31 calories per medium sized fruit, feel free to add a lot of them.

10. Dandelion

Ok, so maybe some of you might say that dandelion grows like a weed around your house. It isn't really exotic, but I've added it here because most people don't think of it as a superfood.

In fact, dandelion has been used for ages as a way to detox the blood and the liver. If taken regularly, it can dissolve kidney stones, prevent liver diseases, cleanse the skin and help clear acne, improve digestion, and stabilize blood sugar. It is rich in beta-carotene and iron.

Dandelion can be taken as a tea or the greens can be cooked as a vegetable. For those who are not used to its taste, it can be a bit bitter. Add a few strips of crumbled bacon to your sauteed greens (you can afford to add this at 23 calories per strip) or add some honey to your tea to minimize the bitterness.

Chapter 3 – Super Grains

Although three of the most popular grain super foods namely, oats, chia, and quinoa are already included in the first two chapters, the other super food grains also deserve to be mentioned. Some are commonly found in the supermarket while others are found in organic or specialty food stores.

1. Buckwheat

Technically and biologically speaking, buckwheat is not a true grain but actually the seed of rhubarb, a broadleaf plant native to the northern parts of Europe and some Asian countries. It is lumped together with all the other grains because of the 'wheat' in its name and because its characteristics are similar to that of the wheat grain. Besides, it is classified as a grain from a culinary perspective because it is cooked similarly as most grains.

Buckwheat origins can be traced back to China. It was widely produced in the country from the 10th to the 13th century A.D. It only spread in Europe and Russia from the 14th to 15th century, and later on n 17th century in the U.S. Today, buckwheat is an essential part of Polish and Russian diets, two countries where this grain is widely produced.

Buckwheat can also be ground into light or dark flour. The darker variety is considered to be more nutritious because it is packed with more nutrients. People with celiac disease or gluten intolerance can safely add buckwheat to their diet because it is gluten-free. In the U.S. alone where there is a high case of celiac disease and gluten intolerance, buckwheat is used as a substitute for wheat products such as pancake batter and bread dough because of its gluten-free property.

Just like the true grains, buckwheat is also rich in fiber, which is why it is extremely helpful if you are planning to lose weight. One cup of buckwheat provides you with almost 20 % of your required daily fiber intake. It also helps manage the blood sugar levels in your body which useful for people with diabetes, helps prevents development of gallstones, keeps blood pressure in check, improves cardiovascular health, and maintains optimum level of cholesterol in your body.

Here are some tips for cooking buckwheat.

- Before cooking buckwheat, you should rinse the grains thoroughly under running water to remove any dust or dirt debris.
- Add one part buckwheat to two parts boiling water. You can also use broth for a more flavorful dish. Turn down the heat when the water with the buckwheat already in it has returned to a boil. Cover the pot with the lid and let it simmer for about half an hour.
- Use buckwheat instead of hot oatmeal for a nutritious breakfast cereal. Eat it with your favorite fruit.
- For a nutritious lunch or dinner, add pumpkin seeds, scallions, garden peas, and chopped chicken to cooked and cooled buckwheat.
- To give your soups and stews a heartier flavor and deeper texture, add cooked buckwheat.

2. Millet

Many people think millet as bird food because it is the main ingredient in bird seed. However, millet is not just bird feed but also a super food because of the many nutrients that it gives to humans. The texture of cooked millet is similar to cooked rice and mashed potatoes because it is both fluffy and creamy.

Millets are tiny, round grains that are available in white, red, yellow, or gray. The most common form of millet available in the supermarket is the hulled millet variety and also couscous made from cracked millet. Millets do not come from a single plant, but from a group of small-seeded grasses grown as cereal crops. They do not belong in a certain taxonomic group but are grouped together according to function. Millets are widely grown in Asia and Africa, usually in developing countries. In fact, 97 % of millet comes from these countries.

Millet is gluten-free and hypoallergenic, perfect for sensitive and allergic people. It is considered a smart carb because it is rich in fiber and has low level of simple sugars which makes it a good grain for diabetic people. It is good for your heart because it lowers the level of cholesterol in your body due to its niacin or vitamin B3 content. It is also easy to digest plus it hydrates your colon which keeps you from being constipated.

To cook millet, you can check out the following tips.

- For basic cooking, rinse the grains to remove dust and dirt and drain. Boil a cup of millet in 2 ½ cups of water. When the mixture is boiling, reduce heat to low, cover the saucepan, and cook for 15 minutes.

Remove from heat and set aside uncovered for about 20 minutes. Add olive oil or butter, and add salt and pepper or herbs to taste.

- You can make it creamier like mashed potatoes by using 3 ½ cups water instead of 2 1/2. Cups. Simmer for 45 minutes to an hour instead of 15 minutes.
- You can also toast millet before cooking for a nuttier flavor. Toast millet in a skillet for about 3 minutes or until fragrant. Be sure to stir constantly to prevent it from burning.
- If you have leftover millet, you can add it in your salads or stir-fried vegetables. You can also simmer it with honey, milk, and cinnamon for a hearty breakfast or shape it into croquettes.

3. Farro

Farro is an ancient variety of wheat which also goes by the name emmer in the U.S., although in Italy, farro refers to three ancient wheat varieties namely, einkorn, spelt, and emmer. Farro is an Italian but is more commonly used to refer to this type of wheat. It is one of the first grains ever farmed by humans for consumption. The composition of ancient wheat such as farro is similar to modern wheat although ancient wheat is generally richer n fiber and protein.

It has a nutty flavor and delicately chewy which tastes a little bit like barley. Farro contains complex carbohydrates that boosts the immune system, lowers cholesterol level, and regulates blood sugar level in the body. It also has antioxidant properties and takes longer to digest which keeps you energized and feeling full for a longer time. Farro is not gluten-free but can help reduce the risks of some cancers, diabetes, and heart disease.

This ancient wheat is popular among chefs because of its versatility. Farro can be served as a delicious and nutritious hot breakfast cereal that you can eat with fruits like peaches, apples, and bananas. There is also one dish called farrotto which is a favorite farro dish cooked like risotto. It can also be a great ingredient for soups, side dishes, and salads. You can also prepare farro as a dessert. Just add a drizzle of honey and a crumbled fresh ricotta cheese.

4. Freekeh

This super grain originated from the Middle East. It is a cereal food that comes from green wheat. Freekeh, sometimes spelled as frikeh, is harvested young, while the seeds are still soft and the grains are still green. Once harvested, it is dried under the sun and undergoes a roasting process to burn the straw and chaff. The seeds are not burned during the roasting process because of the high moisture content. After roasting, the grains still has to undergo another process called thrashing where the grains are rubbed against each other and some more sun-drying to achieve the right color, flavor, and texture. The term freekeh comes from the word *'farik'* which originally means 'rubbed'. They are then cracked into smaller pieces which make them look like green bulgur.

Freekeh is considered as a super grain because it contains more vitamins and minerals compared to other grains. They are also very rich in fiber. In fact, freekeh has four times more fiber than brown rice which makes it a good addition to your weight loss diet. It is also good for digestion because it acts as prebiotic inside the stomach. Prebiotic is the 'food' of good bacteria, and good bacteria improves your digestion. Freekeh is also good for people with diabetes because it has a low glycemic index.

Freekeh is mentioned in an ancient Baghdad cookbook which dates as far back as 13th century. In the old recipe, meat is fried first in oil before braised with water, cinnamon bark, and salt. Freekeh is then added together with dried coriander. The suggested serving is with fresh lamb tail fat, cumin, and cinnamon.

Today, people cook freekeh by adding 2 cups of this ancient grain to 5 cups of cold water and bringing it to a boil. Once it is boiling, reduce the heat and let it simmer for 35 to 40 minutes with the lid on. You can also sprinkle cooked freekeh into salads and soups or mix it with sage, roasted squash, champagne vinegar, and extra virgin olive oil.

5. Amaranth

Amaranth is a close cousin of the more popular super grain quinoa. It was first domesticated 8,000 years ago by the Aztecs who considered it as their staple food. They also used amaranth grains for their religious rituals and ceremonies. However, the cultivation of amaranth stopped when the conquistadores arrived and conquered the Aztec nation. This is the reason why the modern day amaranth has a very similar genetic makeup as the ancient amaranth. In the 1970s, research about the amaranth was conducted and a large tract of land was used for the cultivation of this ancient grain.

Amaranth has high calcium content, which is nearly as much as that of low-fat cottage cheese. It also has higher fiber content, at 5.2 grams per serving, than cold cereals, which have about 1 gram per serving. Compared to a hard-boiled egg, it is also packed with more protein. What sets amaranth apart from other grains is that it contains a type of amino acid called lysine which boosts growth and aids in tissue repair in case of wound or inflammation. People who are suffering from celiac disease and gluten intolerance can add amaranth to their diet because it is gluten-free.

Here are some ways to cook and use amaranth in your meals.

- Boil 3 cups of water or broth with 1 cup of amaranth. After boiling, let it simmer for 20 to 25 minutes with the lid on. Stir occasionally. When amaranth is cooked, the texture and consistency is the same as cooked oatmeal.
- You can use amaranth to whip up healthy breakfast dishes like hot cereal, soup, and porridge.
- Mixing popped amaranth with baked snacks, granola, and mueslis is also a great snack idea.
- Some people also use amaranth as a stuffing to tomatoes and large mushrooms.
- If you are looking for an alternative to wheat flour, you can use amaranth flour when baking.

6. Spelt

Spelt is another really old grain which was cultivated in 5000 BC and was considered a staple food from the Bronze Age to the Middle Ages in some parts of Europe. Today, it is considered as a relict crop and health food in some countries in Europe specifically in northern Spain and Central Europe. It is also a close cousin of the common wheat but is more difficult to buy in local supermarkets. Spelt food products such as flour, pasta, bread, pretzels, biscuits, and pretzels are difficult to buy from local groceries. You need to go to a health food store or specialty bakery.

The nutrients found in this super food are 57.9 % carbohydrates, 17.0 percent protein, 3.0 percent fat, and some vitamins and minerals in smaller amount. It also contains 9.2 percent fiber. Spelt is also used for baking because it contains gluten. This characteristic makes it unsuitable for gluten-free diets for celiacs. Because of the high fiber and protein content of spelt, it helps improve your metabolism which in turn helps you lose weight.

Spelt is used as a substitute for barley and oats in certain food products like cereal, pasta flour, and baked goods. You can add spelt to your diet as a grain or as flour.

Cooking spelt grains is the same as cooking rice by simply boiling it in water. First, rinse the spelt grains in a coriander. Put them in a pot and add water. The ratio of water to spelt is 3:1. Add salt to bring out the flavor of spelt. Bring this to a boil and lower heat once boiling. Leave it to simmer until the grains become tender.

Like farro, you can also cook spelt like risotto. You can add other ingredients you can find in your kitchen such as goat cheese, lemon juice, and fresh greens. Instead of using pasta or rice in your salad, you can use spelt instead for you to enjoy its health benefits. You can also use it when cooking curry with greens.

7. Teff

Most of the super grains in this list are related to the common wheat. Teff, on the other hand, is a member of the lovegrass family and it is the only one that is fully-domesticated. The word 'teff' means 'lost' in Amharic because of the tiny size of the grain which is only less than 1mm in diameter. Teff has long thrived in certain areas of Ethiopia and Eritrea and it has been used by the semi-nomadic people in this area as one of their basic crops. Because of their small size, a handful of teff is enough to plant in a regular-sized field. Their minute size also makes them easy to cook.

Teff contains more calcium than most grains. It has 123 mg of calcium in just one cup, about half as much as a cup of spinach. Vitamin C is present in not commonly found in most grains but teff contains a good amount of this vitamin.

Studies showed that teff is high in resistant starch, a kind of dietary fiber that helps you lose weight, manages blood sugar levels, and boosts colon health.

People in Ehiopia used fermented ground teff flour to make *injera,* a spongy, sourdough bread that is used as an edible serving plate. You can also use teff to make porridge which is a great breakfast dish. It can also be used in pancakes, breads, cereals, snacks, and wraps.

"Dry cook" a cup of teff in one cup water for 6 to 7 minutes then set aside, covered, for another five minutes. The grains will reach the same texture as poppy seeds which make them perfect sprinkles on roasted vegetables or as an addition to soups to give them a creamier texture. You can also cook one cup of teff in 3 cups of water or stock. It is very versatile and can be served boiled, steamed, or baked. You can use teff as an ingredient to your main course or side dish.

Chapter 4 – Super Fruits

Some super fruits have already been included in the first two chapters such as apple, star fruit and different kinds of berries. Just like the super grains, the other super fruits also need to be mentioned because they also help you lose weight and give other health benefits. Here are some popular super fruits that you can add in your weight loss diet plan.

1. Pineapples

Some people do not like pineapples especially when used as toppings on their pizza. However, these tropical fruits are packed with nutrients that your body needs and at the same time help you lose weight. Besides, they are also sweet and juicy that can turn a boring meal into something extraordinary.

Pineapples are made up of coalesced berries, or berries that naturally fused together around a central core to form a single fruit. Pineapples are rich in vitamin C. It also contains vitamins and minerals like manganese and vitamins B1 and B6. It is also rich in fiber which makes it a great fruit for weight loss.

Vitamin C helps boost your immune system by defending all watery areas of the body against the attack of free radicals. Free radicals damage normal cells, which can lead to heart disease, asthma attacks, and cancer, to name a few.

Pineapples are versatile when it comes to cooking and preparation. Peeling and cutting pineapples can be challenging at first but you will get used to it after peeing and cutting a few pineapples.

You can combine pineapples in a variety of dishes. For example, you can mix diced pineapples with shrimp, olive oil, and ginger. Serve this scrumptious salad on a bed of romaine lettuce. You can also prepare salsa using diced pineapple mixed with chili peppers. You can use this salsa to add flavor to different kinds of fish like tuna, halibut, and salmon. Some also serve grilled pineapples while others prepare broiled pineapples with a drizzle of maple syrup then topped with yogurt.

If you are looking for a tasty side dish to chicken, you can mix together chopped pineapples, cashews, and grated fennel. You can also add fresh pineapples to tropical salads that include fruits such as mango, kiwi, and papaya.

2. Bananas

Bananas are the most popular tropical fruit because they are inexpensive and easy to eat. They are full of nutrients yet have low calories which make them a great fruit for those who want to lose weight in a healthy way. The sweet and creamy flesh of bananas also makes them a favorite fruit for breakfast or snack.

Bananas are easy to find because they are available in regular supermarkets. Most bananas have yellow skin but you can also find ripe bananas with green and sometimes even red, purple, pink, and black tones when fully ripe. The different varieties of bananas slightly differ in taste. Some are sweeter while others are starchier. In the United States, the most popular varieties are Cavendish, Martinique, and Big Michael.

Bananas are rich in vitamin B6, vitamin C, manganese, potassium, and fiber. When eaten in moderate amount, bananas are good for your cardiovascular system and digestive system. Endurance athletes also make a habit of eating bananas because of the combination of nutrients that makes them last for hours playing their sport.

Bananas are usually eaten fresh. If you want to cook bananas, you should use plantain bananas which have a starchier quality and are considered more of a vegetable than fruit. Plaintain bananas have higher levels of beta-carotene than other varieties of bananas.

Adults and children love to add peanut butter and a drizzle of honey on their fresh bananas. You can also combine walnuts, chopped bananas, and maple syrup and add the mixture to porridge or oatmeal for a hearty breakfast. For cooking plantain bananas, you can make banana fritters by deep frying sliced plantains coated in a mixture of sugar, flour, and eggs.

3. Oranges

Everyone knows that oranges contain a lot of vitamin C but did you know that they are packed with other nutrients? These round citrus fruits are also rich in fiber, folate, and vitamin B1. They are also a great source of potassium and calcium. Oranges are perfect snacks because they keep you from going hungry until your next meal, which prevents you from eating a lot. They are also used in some recipes that require a tangy flavor. Oranges are considered one of the most popular fruits in the world alongside apples, bananas, and grapes. Oranges are available in your local supermarket year round although the variety differs from season to season.

Because oranges offer a healthy dose of vitamin C, they are considered effective for boosting the immune system and protecting yourself against diseases. Oranges are also great sources of fiber. Fiber boosts the digestive system and reduces level of cholesterol in your bloodstream. It also helps manage the blood sugar level in your body which makes it a perfect snack for people with diabetes. You may not be aware of it but oranges are also beneficial to your kidneys and lungs.

To enjoy the full benefits of oranges, you can eat them fresh or add them in a dish. To prepare an orange sauce, you can sauté onions and ginger. Add the orange juice into the pan. You can use this to complement fish like tuna or salmon.

You can also make a salad by combining fresh orange segments, boiled beets, and fennel. This salad can be a healthy and nutritious side dish.

You can also simmer orange segments, sweet potatoes, and winter squash in orange juice. Sprinkle with walnuts before serving.

4. Avocados

Avocados are also known as alligator pear not because alligators eat them or because they are close cousins of pears but because they are shaped like pears and they have green, leather-like skin that reminds you of alligator skin.

Avocados are rich in pantothenic acid, fiber, vitamin K, and folate. They are also a great source of potassium and vitamins B6, E, and C. Avocados promote good heart health and offer anti-inflammatory benefits. These creamy fruits also promote regulation of blood sugar in your body and helps fight cancer.

Some people think that they should not eat avocados when they are trying to lose weight because these fruits contain more fats than other fruits. However, you need to understand that one cannot get fat by simply eating fat. Avocados contain monosaturated fats which will be provide slow burning fuel for your body. This means that you will have more energy throughout the day even if you just consume a cup of avocado. This will keep you from feeling tired and weak and will make you more physically active. Avocados may have higher calories than other fruits but you will be able to burn them with enough exercise and physical activities.

Monosaturated fats are also helpful in controlling production of insulin and improving glycemic control. These two factors are important if you have diabetes or if you are trying to lose weight.

You can enjoy avocadoes by chopping them and using them as garnish for your black bean soup. You can also turn your simple tofu-based dressing into something richer and creamier by adding chunks of avocado. It will also have that nice green color. Of course, you cannot talk about avocadoes without mentioning guacamoles. To make guacamole, you should mix chopped avocadoes, lime juice, tomatoes, onions, cilantro, and seasoning. You can also make avocado salad by using sliced avocadoes, orange segments, fennel, and mint.

5. Grapefruit

Many people love grapefruit because of its sweet and tangy taste. Just like its cousin the oranges, grapefruits are also juicy and have similar health benefits. Grapefruits are also related to pomelo and lemon. They are available in the groceries all year round but you can find best quality from winter through early spring because they are in season.

Although not as rich in vitamin C as oranges, grapefruits also provide adequate vitamin C that boosts your immune system. They also contain pantothenic acid, fiber, vitamin A, potassium, and vitamin B1. Vitamin C helps treat cold symptoms, which is why you are given fruits that are rich in vitamin C when you have the sniffles. Grapefruit has this nice pink and pink color which is due to a nutrient called lycopene. Lycopene helps fight cancer because they prevent free radicals from attacking and damaging your cells. Keep in mind, though, that white grapefruit does not contain lycopene. Grapefruit also helps lower insulin level which prevents weight gain.

Red and pink grapefruits add a nice color to your green salads. They also provide that tangy spark that makes your salad more appetizing. You can also try drinking a glass of freshly squeezed grapefruit just to add variety to your regular meals. You will find it just as refreshing as your favorite OJ. You can make a salsa by mixing together diced grapefruit, chili peppers, and cilantro. To prepare a scrumptious tropical salad, you can combine chopped grapefruit, avocadoes, and cooked shrimp. Serve the salad on a bed of romaine lettuce.

6. Kiwifruits

Kiwifruit, or more popularly known as kiwi, is native to China and is also called Chinese gooseberry. Missionaries brought these unique fruits to New Zealand in the early 20th century but it was only several decades later when these fruits are commercially grown. In 1961, these fruits were first served in a restaurant in the United States and this was where an American produce distributor discovered the exotic fruit as something that Americans would love in their diet. Because of this, the kiwifruit became known worldwide and is now grown in different countries such as Italy, United States, Japan, Chile, New Zealand, and France.

Kiwi has the same amount of vitamin C as oranges. Unlike other fruits, this exotic fruit (which got its name from the kiwi bird popular in New Zealand because of the skin) also contains vitamin K. It also has vitamin E, potassium, fiber, and folate.

Researchers are fascinated by kiwi's ability to protect the DNA in the human cells, although the exact compound responsible for this benefit is not yet known. Some experts say that it is due to the combinations of carotenoids and flavonoids found in kiwi, although further studies are still required. Kiwi also boosts weight loss because it has fiber. Aside from this, this unique fruit also protects your eyes against macular degeneration and improves your cardiovascular health.

You can eat kiwi fruits as is if you want to fully enjoy their refreshing taste or you can add sliced kiwi in your green salads. You can also prepare a delicious dessert by combining sliced strawberries and kiwi and topping them with yogurt. To prepare chutney which is the perfect side dish for chicken or fish, you can combine sliced kiwi, pineapple, and orange. You probably have not thought of preparing soup using kiwi but this is possible and delicious by blending cantaloupe and kiwi in a blender or food processor. Add yogurt to make it creamier. Some people also use kiwi when making fruit tarts.

7. Apricots

Apricots are those little golden orange fruits with smooth and velvety skin. The fruit has a musky flavor and a tartness that is more noticeable when they are dried. Apricots are closely related to peaches and plums which is why they have similar taste with these fruits.

Apricots are rich in antioxidants which are responsible for the health benefits that they provide. They are also great for people who want to lose weight because they have very few calories. These fruits are also rich in fiber which helps improve your digestion. If you have good digestion, your body will absorb the nutrients from the food that you eat properly and your body will not have a difficult time getting rid of waste products in which in turn helps you lose weight. Apart from this, apricots are also considered as a great source of vitamin A and vitamin C and therefore give you the benefits of these vitamins.

To enjoy apricots, you can add them in your hot or cold cereal for breakfast. You can also mix chopped apricots in your whole grain pancake batter for added flavor and texture. If you are cooking a chicken or vegetable stew, you can give it a Middle Eastern flavor by simply adding diced dried apricots. You can also add fresh apricots to your green salads to give it a sweet and tangy flavor.

8. Plums

These sweet and juicy fruits come in a variety of colors that adding them in your diet will surely make your meals colorful. Believe it or not, plums have over 2,000 different varieties and 100 of them are available in the U.S. They come in different colors such as red, purple, black, yellow, green, orange, green, and different shades of these colors. There are six general categories of plum that you can choose from, namely, American, Damson, Japanese, European/Garden, Ornamental, and Wild. The sizes, shapes, colors, and flesh of these different types of plums vary.

Plums are great sources of vitamin C. They will also help you lose weight because they have the ability to suppress your appetite, which means that you will not get hungry easily after eating them. They also have low calories, about 25 to 30 calories per plum. These amazing fruits also help flush toxic chemicals from your body which helps prevent diseases and they also have anti-inflammatory properties.

Plums are versatile and can be used in a variety of recipes.

- You can broil sliced plums, walnuts, goat cheese, and sage on top of pizza crust or pita bread made of whole wheat.
- You can also poach plums in red wine and serve it with lemon zest for a delicious dessert.
- If you are baking a hardy bread made of rye flour, you can add baked pitted plum halves for added flavor and texture.
- Blended stewed plums are also great for making cold soup, just add honey and yogurt to make it sweeter and creamier.

43

- For an easy and quick breakfast, just add slices of plum to your cold cereal.

You can use different colors of plums with different flavors to add a delightful twist and color to your normal meals.

9. Pears

Pears have different species. Some pear species are cultivated as ornamental trees while others are grown for their juicy and scrumptious fruits. This section will discuss about the edible fruits that help you lose weight and at the same time give you a lot of nutrients that your body needs.

This fruit is a member of the rose family, alongside apples, apricots, plums, and many other fruits. All of the pears that you can find in the supermarket belong to the category European Pear which has a rounded body that tapers near the stem. Pears also come in different colors such as yellow or gold, green, red, and brown. It is difficult to determine ripeness of pears because some species change in color as they ripen.

These sweet and juicy fruits are rich in fiber. It also contains vitamins C and K. Adding pears in your diet will not only make you lose weight but it will also lower your risk of heart disease, diabetes, and cancer because it contains a lot of fiber. Numerous studies already proved that fiber is an essential contributor in fighting these diseases.

You can eat pears by simply peeling the fruits or you can eat the skin as well provided you wash it with clean water thoroughly. You can create a delicious salad by combing chopped pears with watercress, leeks, mustard greens, and walnuts. For a sweet breakfast treat, you can mix together honey, grated ginger, and chopped pears and add the mixture to your porridge made of millet grains. For a scrumptious dessert, you can serve sliced pears topped with bleu or goat cheese. You can also infuse pears with apples juice or wine by simply poaching cored pears into either of these liquids.

Chapter 5 – Vegetable Super Foods

There are many different kinds of vegetables that experts consider as 'super foods'. You might say that everyone already knows that vegetables offer a lot of health benefits. It is a well-known fact even without branding them as super foods. However, there are certain vegetables that are more packed with nutrients than other vegetables plus they also help you lose weight. Here are some super vegetables that you should know about.

1. Tomatoes

Before you react and say that tomatoes are fruits, you first need to hear the explanation why they are included in the vegetables list of super foods. Botanically speaking, tomatoes are fruits but they are considered vegetables from a culinary standpoint and also by the U.S. customs regulations. This is because tomatoes are often prepared and cooked as vegetables rather than fruits.

Whether they are fruits or vegetables, tomatoes are good for your health because they are packed with nutrients that keep you healthy. They are rich in vitamin C and have so many other nutrients which include vitamins K, A, B6, E, and B1 and other nutrients which include but are not limited to potassium fiber, phosphorus, iron, zinc, protein, magnesium, and biotin. Tomatoes also have lycopene, a substance which helps fight cancer. It was found out that lycopene is also present in yellow and tangerine tomatoes, which means that these varieties of tomatoes lower the risk of cancer. Tomatoes are great for people who want to lose weight because they add a sweet flavor to your meals without adding too many calories.

Here are some great ways to enjoy tomatoes:

- Add tomatoes to your bean and vegetable soups.
- Make a salsa dip by combining tomatoes, chili peppers, and onions.
- Prepare a classic Italian salad with mozzarella cheese, onions, and tomatoes drizzled with olive oil.
- Blend cucumbers, bell peppers, scallions, and tomatoes in a food processor until the mixture reaches a smooth texture. Season with herbs and spices and use this to make a delightful cold soup or gazpacho.
- Add tomato slices to your salads and sandwiches to give them that fresh and juicy flavor. You can even use different colors of tomatoes such as red, green, and yellow to make your salads more colorful.

2. Broccoli

It is a well-known fact that broccoli is good for your health. However, this is one of the vegetables that kids don't like. You probably didn't like broccoli as a child but it turns out that your parents are correct. You should eat more of these vegetables because they are considered super foods which mean that they are rich in nutrients.

For people who want to lose weight, broccoli is a great vegetable because it makes you feel full plus it is rich in fiber which makes you feel good because you do not have any problems with your bowel movement. Broccoli also helps lower your cholesterol level, especially when they are steamed. Fresh broccoli also has this ability but not as much as steamed broccoli.

These vegetables boost your body's detoxification system because it contains phytonutrients. Broccoli also has vitamins A and K which are essential in solving vitamin C deficiencies. Aside from these benefits, this amazing vegetable also has flavonoid which is responsible broccoli's anti-inflammatory and hypoallergenic properties.

You can serve broccoli in a variety of ways such as the ones listed below.

- Add steamed broccoli florets, pine nuts, olive oil, and pasta. Toss the ingredients together and season with salt and pepper.
- To make a delicious soup, puree cooked cauliflower and broccoli in a food processor and season with herbs and spices.
- When making omelets, add chopped florets and stalks of broccoli to add texture and turn it into a healthier breakfast.

Broccolis are versatile and can be served fresh, steamed, or stir-fried or you can cook it as ingredients in a dish.

3. Spinach

Spinach is a popular vegetable that you will usually see on the plates of children whose parents make an effort to provide them with healthy and nutritious meals. It is also popular because Popeye eats spinach and everyone who grew up watching this cartoon show knows how his muscles grow and how he becomes really strong after eating spinach. Although you will not get that kind of muscle by eating spinach alone and you will not see the positive result as quickly, you will surely enjoy a number of healthy benefits when you add spinach to your diet. For instance, spinach has anti-cancer and anti-inflammatory properties. It also helps you maintain good bone health. It is good for people who are on a weight loss diet plan because it makes you feel full without adding too much calories.

Spinach originated in the Middle East, specifically in ancient Persia or what is known now as modern Iran and some nearby countries. This leafy vegetable was brought to India by Arab traders, then to ancient China. In AD 827, spinach was brought to Sicily, which makes the vegetable a part of the Mediterranean cuisine. Ever since it was brought to Europe, the popularity of this vegetable started to spread in other countries such as Spain, Germany, England, and France. In fact, queen Catherine de' Medici of France used to love spinach so much that she always had it served in her every meal. This is the reason why dishes with spinach are called 'Florentine' as a tribute to queen Catherine who was born in Florence, France.

Green leafy vegetables such as spinach are rich in iron. This vegetable is also a great source of antioxidants and vitamins A, C, E, K, B2, and B6. It also contains magnesium, manganese, folate, potassium and folic acid, to list down a few nutrients. You will still get the antioxidants whether the spinach is fresh, quickly boiled, or steamed. However, some of nutrients such as folate will be reduced if you boil the spinach.

Here are a few quick serving ideas for spinach.

- Add several layers of spinach when you cook lasagna.

- To add crunch to your cooked spinach, you can add pine nuts to it.
- For your side dish or even a light meal, you can prepare spinach with tomatoes and cheese.

4. Asparagus

Asparagus is a close relative of onions and garlic and is considered a spring vegetable. It is native to most countries in Europe, western Asia, and northern Africa. This perennial crop is not just considered as a vegetable but also as a medicine. It has diuretic properties, which means that asparagus promotes the excretion of water from the body such as urine. This is helps treat heart failure, kidney problems, liver cirrhosis, and hypertension. Asparagus also has a very delicate flavor which makes it a great addition to many different kinds of dishes. Some people also eat it fresh such as in salads or as a snack.

Asparagus makes you feel full without adding too many calories because it is composed of 93 % water. It also contains vitamins and minerals such as calcium, zinc, vitamin K, vitamin B6, and magnesium. Asparagus also has vitamins C, E, and K which provides different health benefits such as stronger immune system, healthier skin, and stronger bones.

You need to know that only young asparagus shoots are used for culinary purposes because they are still tender and at the same time crunchy. When the buds star to open, the stalk or shoot will turn hard or woody, which makes it difficult to bite or chew. It is also becomes a little drier and no longer good for cooking. Asparagus is considered a luxury vegetable because it is more expensive than other vegetables. There are

50

three varieties of asparagus that are available in the supermarket—green, white, and purple asparagus. These three varieties differ in taste. For example, white asparagus has a more delicate flavor and tender texture and is usually sold in cans, although you can find some fresh white asparagus in gourmet stores. White asparagus is more expensive than the other two because it is more difficult to grow and produce. Purple asparagus is smaller but has a fruitier flavor. Green asparagus is the most common type and can easily be found in regular supermarkets.

You can enjoy asparagus in a number of ways.

- Add chopped asparagus to your omelets to add flavor and color.
- Sauté garlic, shiitake mushrooms, and asparagus, then add tofu or chicken for a healthy main dish.
- Turn your simple green salad into something more luxurious by adding cold chopped asparagus.
- Mix together olive oil, pasta spices, and asparagus and toss freshly cooked pasta with the mixture. You can use a combination of rosemary, tarragon, and thyme for your pasta spices or you can choose other herbs that you like.

5. Kale

Kale used to be one of the most popular green vegetables in Europe until the end of the medieval era. It was in the 19th century when kale was introduced to Canada, then later on to the U.S. by Russian traders. Even before, people already understood the nutritional value of Kale. For instance, kale was widely cultivated in the UK during World War II because it is easy to grow and soldiers can still get important nutrients despite having to eat ration meals.

Kale has beautiful green or purple leaves which are the ones used for cooking. It is a close cousin of cauliflower, broccoli, Brussels sprouts, and collard greens. It has an earthy flavor that gives dishes a distinct taste and even though it is packed with nutrients, you do not have to worry about gaining weight because kale has fewer calories than other foods. Although kale is available in groceries all year round, this leafy vegetable is in season from the middle of winter to early spring, which means that they have the sweetest taste and are more widely available during this period.

The most common varieties of kale are ornamental kale or salad savoy, curly kale, and dinosaur kale. These different varieties slightly differ in appearance, texture, and taste. When buying kale from the supermarket, you need to choose the ones that have firm and deeply colored leaves and have hardy yet moist stem. If the leaves are already wilted and have started to turn brown or yellow, you should skip this because it means that it is no longer fresh.

The healthiest way to cook kale is to steam it for 5 minutes for you to get the maximum taste and flavor. You can toss it with Mediterranean dressing and add some of your favorite vegetables. To enjoy kale, you can braise chopped kale and apples and sprinkle with chopped walnuts and balsamic vinegar before serving. You can also use combine feta cheese, pine nuts, and chopped kale and toss with whole grain pasta with olive oil.

6. Arugula

People also call this leafy green 'salad rocket' from the French word *roquette* which is also another nickname for this plant. Arugula is a member of the brassicaceae family, alongside cauliflower, kale, cabbage, and mustard greens, and is considered an early summer vegetable. Arugula has a lot of health benefits which you might not expect from something that looks small and delicate. Here are some health benefits of arugula.

- Arugula helps people maintain their ideal weight because it has fewer calories than other vegetables but it has loads of flavor that does not make you feel as if you are always eating bland meals. This prevents you from feeling deprived because you can still eat flavorful dishes.
- You can get a lot of nutrients from arugula such as vitamins A, C, and K plus it also has folic acid. Only a few vegetables have vitamin K, which is known for improving bone health and boosts brain power.
- This zippy veggie is rich in phytochemicals which can help fight cancer by protecting your body from free radicals that cause damage to your cells.
- Spinach may be the best source of iron among the leafy greens but arugula comes in close second. It has higher levels of iron and copper which is important for nutrient absorption.
- This summer vegetable is perfect for the season because of its peppery flavor which has a refreshing and cooling effect on your body. It also has high water content which makes your body hydrated during the hot summer weather. This is the perfect food for summer picnics.

- Arugulas are also considered aphrodisiac because it has a stimulating effect on the body which keeps you more active and energized.

To enjoy arugula, you can combine with other greens for a healthy green salad. Some European countries also use fresh arugula to add flavor to pasta and meat dishes. When preparing pizza, you can add arugula immediately after baking or before the baking ends to prevent it from wilting. You can also make a sauce by frying arugula in olive oil and garlic which adds flavor to fish and cold meats.

7. Mushrooms

This is the only one in the list which does not belong to the plant kingdom. Mushrooms are not true vegetables but are considered vegetables from a culinary standpoint. Biologically speaking, mushrooms are not vegetables because they are not members of the plant kingdom. For those who are not familiar with the biological makeup of mushrooms, these are edible fungi. Yes, they belong in the same categories as yeast and those fungi that cause disease. But of course, these edible mushrooms are safe to eat and are in fact delicious. However, mushrooms are considered vegetables by chefs and cooks because they are cooked and prepared in the same way as vegetables, not fruits.

Mushrooms are usually used in Asian cuisines. Western people especially Americans have just started to appreciate the flavor and texture of these edible fungi and slowly incorporate them in their traditional dishes. Mushrooms are ideal for people who want to lose weight because they are low in fat and sodium. They also provide wonderful flavors to your dishes such because it contains glutamic acid, a natural flavor enhancer which you can also find in MSG or monosodium glutamate that gives your dishes that *umami* or savory taste.

These 'vegetables' are also perfect for vegetarians because they have similar nutrients as meat. For example, they can be a source of protein when cooked. It may not provide you with your full protein requirement but this can easily be solved by adding grains to your diet. Aside from protein, mushrooms also have iron, niacin, and riboflavin. They are also rich in fiber. Always stick to cooked mushrooms because they provide up to 4x more nutrients than raw mushrooms.

It is important not to wash the mushrooms when cleaning them because they absorb water like sponge. You can clean them by using a special brush for mushroom or by using a slightly damp cloth. They can add flavor to your soup by throwing in the trimmed stems of the mushrooms. You can also sauté mushrooms with garlic and onion and some seasoning. Cook them in a small drizzle of vegetable oil with wine. You also need to remember that mushrooms add liquid to your dishes so do not add as much water if you are using mushrooms as ingredients.

8. Cabbage

Cabbage is related to other cole vegetables such as Brussels sprouts, cauliflower, and broccoli. You can find green cabbage and purple cabbage, although green cabbage is more common. Cabbage plants are grown for their round heads which are composed of dense leaves. The inner leaves of the cabbages are usually light in color because they are not exposed to the sun. These cruciferous vegetables are abundant and inexpensive which makes them a dietary staple in different countries throughout the world and are available all year round because they store really well, although they are in season from late fall through winter season.

This vegetable is used both as food and medicine. According to history, Celtic wanderers brought wild cabbage to Europe in 600 B.C. In fact, ancient Roman and Greek civilizations regard cabbage as a really effective plant medicine that treats a variety of illnesses. Countries across Europe, Japan, and China are the top considered the top producers of cabbage in the world today.

Cabbages are rich in vitamins K and C which are known for improving bone health and immune system, respectively. They are also great sources of vitamin B6, fiber, and manganese. They have anti-cancer and anti-inflammatory benefits. Cabbage has no fat or cholesterol and has very low calories, which makes them a great addition to your weight loss meals.

There are a number of ways to enjoy the nutritious benefits of cabbage.

- You can make sauerkraut which is a famous German dish by fermenting finely cut cabbage. Sauerkraut literally means 'sour cabbage'. Because this is fermented, it has a long shelf life. You can use sauerkraut as a condiment for hot dogs and various meat dishes.
- You can braise chopped red cabbage, chopped apples, and red wine.
- You can also mix together both red and green cabbage and add olive oil, fresh lemon juice, and some spices like cumin, coriander, black pepper, and turmeric for a delicious Indian coleslaw.

9. Carrots

Bug Bunny loves them and it is no wonder why. Carrots are crunchy and crisp when fresh. They also have a sweet taste that makes them great ingredients for desserts like carrot cakes. The history of this orange root crop can be traced back thousands of years ago. The ancient carrot was originally cultivated in Middle Eastern, Central Asian, and some European countries. These look slightly different from the modern orange carrots because they come in unusual colors like yellow, red, and purple. These hardy vegetables were brought to America during the 15th to 16 centuries. Today, the top producers of carrots are China, Russia, and the U.S. The U.S. alone is a major consumer of carrots. An average adult eats about 12 pounds of carrots in just one year or about 1 cup of carrot a week.

Everyone knows that carrots are rich in vitamin A, which is why they are good for the eyes. They also have an abundant supply of antioxidant such as beta-carotene and other types of antioxidants. These help improve cardiovascular healthy and helps prevent cancer. Carrots are also great vegetables if you are trying to lose weight because one serving only has 50 calories.

When buying carrots from the supermarket, you have to check if they are firm and smooth and if the color is still bright orange because carrots with deeper orange colors means they have more beta-carotene. If stored properly, carrots will last for a longer time than other vegetables. You can store them in a plastic bag before putting them inside the fridge.

Here are a few fast and easy serving ideas for these delightful orange vegetables.

- You can add chopped fresh carrots to salads.
- You can shred carrots and combine them with apples and beets for a fresh and tasty salad.
- You can also puree boiled potatoes and carrots in a food processor and season with your favorite herbs and spices for a hearty and nutritious soup.
- Instead of serving chips and dips at parties, you should instead serve spiced carrot sticks. To do this, you need to heat water with coriander seeds, cayenne, and salt. Soak the carrot sticks into the hot mixture. Set aside to cool before draining. Serve to your guests.

10.   Leeks

Leeks are cousins of onions, garlic, scallions, and shallots. They have a very small bulb and a long white stalk with layers of green, flat leaves tightly wrapped around the stalk. They resemble large scallions in physical appearance but they taste more like shallots, only a little sweeter and with a less intense flavor. There are also wild leeks called ramps that are smaller and has a stronger flavor than cultivated leeks. Leeks grow for a short period of time every year and they are widely sought out by buyers at supermarkets when they are in season.

Leeks are rich in vitamin K and manganese and are a decent source of vitamin B6, iron, vitamin C, vitamin A, and fiber. Because they are rich in fiber, leeks help regulate your bowel movement and treat constipation, which makes you feel good. They also help cleanse the digestive tract by getting rid of accumulated remnant of food in your body, which means that it also aids in your body's detoxification. It is a potent laxative which keeps your stomach clean and this in turn helps you lose weight.

The healthiest way to cook leek is by heating 3 tablespoons of broth in a skillet and adding a pound of cut leek into the skillet. Cover for four minutes. Add a couple more tablespoons of broth and bring heat to low. Saute for 3 more minutes without the cover. Stir frequently. Toss with 1 teaspoon of lemon juice, 2 tablespoon of olive oil, and season with salt and pepper.

Another way to enjoy leeks is by sautéing chopped leeks with fennel. Add lemon juice and thyme as garnish. To give your salad that sweet taste, you can add finely chopped leeks. You can also make a cold soup called vichyssoise by blending together cooked potatoes and leeks in a food processor until they reach the consistency of a puree. Finally, you can add leeks to stews and broth to give them a nice flavor.

Chapter 6 – Meat and Poultry

Some people may think that super foods for weight loss only include vegetables, fruits, grains, fish, and those other foods that are packed with nutrients but low in calorie or at least help you flush out unwanted food remnants from your body. However, you will be surprised to note that meat and poultry can also be considered as super foods that help you lose weight as long as you choose only the highest quality and you eat them in moderation. These may not be suitable for those who are planning to go vegetarian but these are great protein sources for people who are trying to lose weight but do not necessarily want to eliminate meat from their diet.

1. Chicken breast

Many people who go on a diet and who want to build muscles like body builders opt for chicken breasts when it comes to their source of protein. Chicken breasts have high protein content but low in fat. This is considered high quality protein and is one of the most popular meats in the U.S. You will find a lot of American meals that have chicken in them.

The most important thing is to always choose skinless chicken breasts because chicken skin is high in fat. It is also best to cook it in a grill with herbs and spices than to coat it with breading because breading will only add up to your total calorie intake.

When you eat grilled chicken breast, you will feel full without having to worry about extra calories. A 3-ounce serving of chicken breast without bone and skin only gives you 102 calories. Fried chicken, even if it is chicken breast, is a big no-no if you are on a diet because it contains a lot more calories plus they also have unhealthy fats. The same amount of chicken breast gives you 19 grams of quality protein. Protein is important for people who are trying to lose weight because it makes them feel full and at the same time helps them burn calories and lose fat because they fell more energetic. Improving your dietary protein intake also boosts your body composition, which means that you will lose fat and increase lean body mass. It also helps increase your body's energy expenditure while working out or dong physical activities.

You can grill chicken breast after coating it with your favorite spices. You can also bake it by preheating oven to 350 degrees for up to 20 to 25 minutes. You can add salsa made from healthy herbs and vegetables to your chicken breast before baking. Some of the liquid will evaporate once the chicken starts to bake. You can also use thicker sauces like barbecue or ranch dressing but be sure to add a little water or broth to prevent it from sticking into the baking pan, then drain the sauce afterwards.

2. Organic lean meat

Lean meats have less fat than regular meat which makes them a great source of protein for people who are on a diet. However, you have to make sure that you are buying organic lean meat and not those commercially produced lean meat because commercial farms that grow cows, pigs, and other animals for human consumption usually pump antibiotics and growth hormones to these animals to make them extraordinarily big so that they will produce bigger and thicker slabs of meat. And of course, you do not want these kinds of meat in your diet not only because they will thwart your weight loss efforts but also because they can cause more harm than good to your health.

Organic lean meats may have the same nutrients as regular commercial meats but they surely do not have those chemicals that can put your health at risk. Organic lean meats, or anything organic for that matter, may be more expensive than other conventional counterparts but at least you know that you are not eating anything artificial. If you cannot find organic lean meats, you can at least go with all-natural or grass-fed lean meat.

Grilled lean meat is still the best method of cooking meat to give it that nice smoky flavor. You can also bake it if you like. Just season the meat a little bit with your favorite herbs and spices.

3. Turkey Breast

All the parts of turkey are virtually carbohydrate-free but the breast has the lowest calorie and fat contents. For instance, a serving or 3 ounce of roasted turkey breast has 6 grams of fat, 24 grams of protein, and 160 calories.

It is easy to include turkey in your weight loss diet plan because you can use it as an alternative to chicken. For example, instead of eating a regular hamburger which is loaded with fats and calories, you should instead prepare a grilled turkey burger for your meal. Just make sure that you buy at least 90 % lean ground turkey. You can also switch from your regular ham sandwich to turkey sandwich, chili with ground turkey instead of ground beef, or use small pieces of turkey breast in your stir-fried dishes.

4. Eggs

Eggs are included in this chapter because they are related to poultry. Eggs are a subject of debate among weight loss experts. Some say it helps you lose weight while other say it only makes you gain weight. However, studies show that eating eggs does not necessarily make one lose or gain weight, although eggs contain protein that helps you curb your appetite and makes you feel more energetic which allows you to do more physical activities and workouts.

When choosing eggs, it is important to buy organic, pasture-raised eggs from local farms or organic stores. It is best to buy organic eggs because they usually have higher nutrient quality and choosing organic also reduces the risk of contamination. When you shop for eggs, you will find out that there are so many labels describing eggs such as cage-free, free-range, pastured, and pasture-raised. Pasture-raised eggs are the best choice because they have better nutrient quality and higher levels of certain vitamins and minerals. Pasture-raised eggs come from chickens that are raised out into the pasture and allowed to forage on legumes and grasses. Some studies say that these eggs have 200 % more vitamins than chickens grown inside cages.

It is widely known that eggs are a great source of high-quality protein. If you are trying to lose weight, your body still needs protein and it is important to get only the best quality, such as the protein found in eggs. Protein from eggs is used as the standard for food proteins from other food sources. Eggs also have a variety of B vitamins and the one that stands out is choline, which is an important nutrient to keep your cells healthy.

When you buy eggs from the supermarket, they are usually lumped together with dairy products because they all come from animals. However, you need to understand that eggs have a different nutritional makeup than dairies. The most common type of eggs is chicken eggs, although you can also buy eggs from other bird species like ducks and quail eggs. No matter what type of eggs you bought, they have the same two basic components—the yolk and the white. The white contains 87 % water and 13 % protein, while the yolk has 50 % water, 17 % protein, and 33 % fat. Some diet plans ban egg yolks because of the fat content. However, as long as you eat in moderation, have a balanced diet, and get enough exercise, you can add yolks in your diet.

You can eat plain hard-boiled eggs or you can chop it and add leeks, dill, fresh lemon juice and olive oil for a healthy salad. You can also make Egg Benedict by preparing an English muffin, lining it with steamed spinach, and placing the poached egg on top.

Chapter 7 – Drinks

Lastly, we arrive at the superfood drinks. Depending on where you are, some of these may be found in your supermarket or else, like in the case of aloe vera, you can grow them yourself.

1. Coconut water

Coconut water is the water found inside the coconut. This is different from coconut cream or milk which comes from squeezing the grated coconut milk.

Though coconut water has been a refreshing tropical treat since the beginning of time, celebrities like Madonna have made it famous in the West. It is low in calories and high in electrolytes thus making it a great alternative for those fancy sports drinks created for athletes. It can also ease a hangover, reduce acid reflux and prevent constipation.

Though you might be tempted to add sugar to coconut water, it is better to drink it as is. Coconut water is sold in tetra packs or bottles, but if you find an Asian market which sells fresh coconuts, try to get it there to ensure the freshest possible product.

2. Tea

Most people are already familiar with the health benefits of tea. Whether you choose black, green, oolong or puerh tea, you get a ton of antioxidants and a boost in weight loss from the thermogenesis effect. Research suggests that regularly drinking tea makes your body burn more calories throughout the day even at rest.

This is not to say that tea can replace regular exercise, but when it comes to weight loss every calorie burn counts. Tea can also make you cut back on too much snacking. If you are plagued by emotional eating, a hot cup of unsweetened or slightly sweetened tea will make you feel as if you have eaten something.

If you don't like hot drinks, you can still get the benefits of tea even if it is cold. Make a batch of iced tea and keep it in the fridge for a refreshing drink. Mix it with lemonade, pulverized fruits or herbal teas to alter the flavor.

3. Yerba mate tea

This is a type of South American herbal tea which is made from the leaves of the mate tree. Like tea, it contains antioxidants and a slight amount of caffeine. It also gives a thermogenesis effect which can help with weight loss.

It might be a bit of an acquired taste for those who are more used to the taste of tea. If you wish to follow tradition, get yourself a metal straw which is traditionally used when drinking yerba mate tea.

4. Chrysanthemum tea

This is another kind of herbal tea made from dried chrysanthemum flowers. It tastes very flowery and is great when mixed with a little honey. This tea has been used in China to cure headaches, skin ailments, and anxiety. It looks extremely pretty too since the hot water makes the dried flowers open up as if in bloom.

Drinking a lot of liquids is good for weight loss because it fills up your stomach without giving you too many calories. As such, chrysanthemum tea is a great alternative for the other teas listed above.

5. Rose hip tea

Rose hip tea is another kind of herbal tea which is reported to be good for the skin. It contains a high level of vitamin C and tastes sweet and flowery. You don't have to add any sweeteners to this for it to taste good. Some people like to add this to black or green tea to avoid the need to add sweeteners. This can also be added to lemonade, mixed with chrysanthemum tea or steeped in milk.

6. Aloe vera gel

Aloe vera gel has a multitude of purposes from curing skin ailments to soothing burns to weight loss. Regarding the last purpose, the gel has a mild laxative effect which helps to prevent you from being bloated.

Make sure that you buy aloe vera gel that is fit for consumption. Those used for topical purposes might be mixed with preservatives or moisturizers. You can also buy an aloe vera plant and harvest the gel yourself. If you water your plant regularly and keep it in the sun, you will never run out of aloe vera gel.

The best way to consume aloe vera gel is to combine it with cold juice or smoothies.

7. Wine

Wine contains a significant amount of antioxidants which can improve heart health if taken in reasonable amounts. Further, scientists have discovered that a daily glass of wine can make your body burn more calories due to a thermogenesis effect just like with tea and yerba mate tea.

That said, take note that too much wine can stimulate your appetite and make you eat more. Make sure that you limit yourself to only a glass or two of wine and drink tea for the rest of the day.

8. Vinegar

Though it seems unappetizing, drinking vinegar will improve your digestion and lower the Glycemic Index of refined carbohydrates. It has been proven that taking vinegar with white carbohydrates like bread, pasta and potatoes will prevent the blood sugar from spiking.

If this has made you wrinkle your nose, you will be happy to know that you are not supposed to drink vinegar by the glass-full. You can get the health benefits of vinegar by taking only a tablespoon or by adding it to your dishes. Splash some vinegar on your fries, or serve bread like the Italians do with a dip of olive oil and balsamic vinegar.

Chapter 8 – How to Eat "the Superfoods"

There are 60 superfoods listed in this book, but other sources might give you even more. With so much to choose from, it might get a bit confusing how you are supposed to eat all these.

The truth is you don't have to eat all of these superfoods all the time. Remember that the basics of good nutrition still apply here. Any food consumed in excess will be bad for you. You should try to vary your diet as much as possible so you will get all the health benefits without numbing your taste buds from repetitiveness.

For example, you can eat oranges for their vitamin C, then alternate them with rosehip tea or camu camu juice. You can eat plain oatmeal today and mix them with chia seeds the next. You can add goji berries to your morning tea then eat them as a snack later in the afternoon.

Also, don't feel bad if you are not able to obtain the exotic choices listed above. Oatmeal can provide you with fiber if you cannot buy quinoa, and strawberries can be as good as star fruit in your fruit salad.

Conclusion

Thank you again for purchasing this book!

I hope this book was able to help you to know the superfoods which help to maintain good health and encourage your weight loss.

The next step is to check your local market for what is available and plan your meals with these superfoods.

Finally, if you enjoyed this book, please take the time to share your thoughts and post a review on Amazon. We do our best to reach out to readers and provide the best value we can. Your positive review will help us achieve that. It'd be greatly appreciated!

Thank you and good luck!

Check Out My Other Books

Below you'll find some of my other popular books that are popular on Amazon and Kindle as well. Simply click on the links below to check them out. Alternatively, you can visit my author page on Amazon to see other work done by me.

Coconut Oil for Easy Weight Loss: A Step by Step Guide for Using Virgin Coconut Oil for Quick and Easy Weight Loss

http://www.amazon.com/Coconut-Oil-Easy-Weight-Loss-ebook/dp/B00JG8H8DE

Carrier Oils for Beginners: Discover the Characteristics and Beauty and Health Benefits of Carrier Oils For mixing Aromatherapy Essential Oils

http://www.amazon.com/Carrier-Oils-Beginners-Characteristics-Aromatherapy-ebook/dp/B00K88GI2S

Natural Homemade Cleaning Recipes For Beginners: Essential Oil Recipes For Household Cleaning, Laundry & Toxic Free Living

http://www.amazon.com/Natural-Homemade-Cleaning-Recipes-Beginners-ebook/dp/B00K87UBQI

The Best Secrets of Natural Remedies: The Ultimate Guide to Natural Remedies to Prevent and Cure Illnesses, Cold and Flu for Your Family

http://www.amazon.com/Best-Secrets-Natural-Remedies-Illnesses-ebook/dp/B00JNDCOCM

The Hypothyroidism Handbook:An Everyday Guide to Natural Solutions of living with Hypothyroidism including increased energy, lasting weight loss, and general well-being

http://www.amazon.com/Hypothyroidism-Handbook-Solutions-including-increased-ebook/dp/B00JNIGIV0

The Hyperthyroidism Handbook: An Everyday Guide to Natural Solutions of Living with Hyperthyroidism including Weight Gain, Increased Energy and General Well-being

http://www.amazon.com/Hyperthyroidism-Handbook-Solutions-including-Hypothyroidism-ebook/dp/B00JOHU5SM

Essential Oils & Weight Loss for Beginners: Ultimate Guide to Losing Weight, Increasing Energy, Balancing Metabolism & Appetite Using Essential Oils & Aromatherapy

http://www.amazon.com/Essential-Oils-Weight-Loss-Beginners-ebook/dp/B00JOFOWP6

Top Essential Oil Recipes: A Recipe Guide Of Natural, Non-Toxic Aromatherapy & Essential Oils for Healing Common Ailments, Beauty, Stress & Anxiety

http://www.amazon.com/Top-Essential-Oil-Recipes-Aromatherapy-ebook/dp/B00JY434E2

Soap Making For Beginners: A Guide to Making Natural Homemade Soaps from Scratch, Includes Recipes and Step by Step Processes for Making Soaps

http://www.amazon.com/Soap-Making-Beginners-Homemade-Processes-ebook/dp/B00JYKH75I

Body Butters For Beginners: Proven Secrets To Making All Natural Body Butters For Rejuvenating And Hydrating Your Skin

http://www.amazon.com/Body-Butters-Beginners-Rejuvenating-Hydrating-ebook/dp/B00K6LVV6A

Apple Cider Vinegar For Beginners: Proven Secrets Using Apple Cider Vinegar For Health, Weight Loss, and Skin Care

http://www.amazon.com/Apple-Cider-Vinegar-Beginners-Aromatherapy-ebook/dp/B00K6YY6HI

Homemade Body Scrubs & Masks For Beginners: 50 Proven All Natural, Easy Recipes For Body & Facial Masks To Exfoliate Nourish, & Care For Your Skin

http://www.amazon.com/Homemade-Body-Scrubs-Masks-Beginners-ebook/dp/B00K79D4SY

Essential Oils Box Set #1: Essential Oils & Weight Loss For Beginners (Ultimate Guide to Losing Weight, Increasing Energy, Balancing Metabolism & Appetite Using Essential Oils & Aromatherapy) + Top Essential Oil Recipes (A Recipe Guide of Natural, Non-Toxic Aromatherapy & Essential Oils for Healing Common Ailments, Beauty, Stress & Anxiety)

http://www.amazon.com/ESSENTIAL-OILS-BOX-SET-Aromatherapy-ebook/dp/B00K7Q8HRK

Essential Oils Box Set #2: Essential Oils & Weight Loss For Beginners (Ultimate Guide to Losing Weight, Increasing Energy, Balancing Metabolism & Appetite Using Essential Oils & Aromatherapy) + Top Essential Oil Recipes (A Recipe

Guide of Natural, Non-Toxic Aromatherapy & Essential Oils for Healing Common Ailments, Beauty, Stress & Anxiety)

http://www.amazon.com/ESSENTIAL-OILS-BOX-SET-Aromatherapy-ebook/dp/B00K7Q8HRK

Box Set#3: Coconut Oil for Easy Weight Loss(A Step by Step Guide for Using Virgin Coconut Oil for Quick and Easy Weight Loss) + Apple Cider Vinegar(Proven Secrets Using Apple Cider Vinegar for Health, Weight Loss, and Skin Care)

http://www.amazon.com/Box-Set-Beginners-Aromatherapy-Essential-ebook/dp/B00K9TEGUW

Box Set #4: Body butters For Beginners(Proven Secrets To Making All Natural Body Butters For Rejuvenating And Hydrating Your Skin) & Top Essential Oil Recipes: A Recipe Guide Of Natural, Non-Toxic Aromatherapy & Essential Oils for Healing Common Ailments, Beauty, Stress & Anxiety

http://www.amazon.com/Box-Set-Butters-Beginners-Essential-ebook/dp/B00KA02F4Y

Box Set #5: Soap Making For Beginners(A Guide to Making Natural Homemade Soaps from Scratch, Includes Recipes and Step by Step Processes for Making Soaps) + Homemade Body Scrubs & Masks For Beginners(50 Proven All Natural, Easy Recipes For Body Scrub & Facial Masks To Efoliate, Nourish, & Care For Your Skin)

http://www.amazon.com/Box-Set-Beginners-Homemade-Recipes-ebook/dp/B00K9U3I2I

Box Set #6: Body Butters for Beginners (Proven Secrets To Making All Natural Body Butters For Rejuvenating And Hydrating Your Skin) +Homemade Body Scrubs & Masks For Beginners(50 Proven All Natural, Easy Recipes For Body Scrub & Facial Masks To Exfoliate, Nourish, & Care For Your Skin)

http://www.amazon.com/Box-Set-Beginners-Exfoliating-Moisturizing-ebook/dp/B00K9U3Y4O

Box Set #7: TOP ESSENTIAL OILS(A Recipe Guide Of Natural, Non-Toxic Aromatherapy & Essential Oils For Healing, Common Ailments, Beauty, Stress & Anxiety) & THE BEST SECRETS OF NATURAL REMEDIES(The Ultimate Guide to Natural Remedies to Prevent and Cure Illnesses, Cold and Flu for Your Family)

http://www.amazon.com/BOX-SET-Essential-Recipes-Remedies-ebook/dp/B00K9WPMQG

Box Set #8: NATURAL HOMEMADE CLEANING RECIPES FOR BEGINNERS (Essential Oil Recipes for Household Cleaning, Laundry & Toxic Free Living) + TOP ESSENTIAL OILS(A Recipe Guide Of Natural, Non-Toxic Aromatherapy & Essential Oils For Healing, Common Ailments, Beauty, Stress & Anxiety)

http://www.amazon.com/BOX-SET-Beginners-Essential-Aromatherapy-ebook/dp/B00KAMNGBS

Box Set #9: Essential Oils & Weight Loss for Beginners (Ultimate Guide to Losing Weight, Increasing Energy, Balancing Metabolism & Appetite Using Essential Oils & Aromatherapy) + Carrier Oils for Beginners (Discover the

Characteristics and Beauty and Health Benefits of Carrier Oils for Mixing Aromatherapy Essential Oils)

http://www.amazon.com/BOX-SET-Essential-Beginners-Aromatherapy-ebook/dp/B00KAODL6Q

BOX SET #10: THE HYPERTHYROIDISM HANDBOOK (An Everyday Guide to Natural Solutions of Living with Hyperthyroidism including Weight Gain, Increased Energy and General Well-being) + THE HYPOTHYROIDISM HANDBOOK (Everyday Guide to Natural Solutions of Living With Hypothyroidism Including Increased Energy, Lasting Weight Loss, and General Well-Being)

http://www.amazon.com/BOX-SET-10-Hyperthyroidism-Hypothyroidism-ebook/dp/B00KAKMSBY

BOX SET #11: CARRIER OILS FOR BEGINNERS (Discover the Characteristics and Beauty and Health Benefits of Carrier Oils for Mixing Aromatherapy Essential Oils) + Essential Oils & Aromatherapy for Beginners (Secrets to Beauty, Health and Weight Loss Using Proven Essential Oil and Aromatherapy Recipes

http://www.amazon.com/BOX-SET-Beginners-Essential-Aromatherapy-ebook/dp/B00KAONEQ8

BOX SET 12: ESSENTIAL OILS & WEIGHT LOSS FOR BEGINNERS: (Ultimate Guide to Losing Weight, Increasing Energy, Balancing Metabolism & Appetite Using Essential Oils & Aromatherapy) + TOP ESSENTIAL OIL RECIPES (A Recipe Guide of Natural, Non-Toxic Aromatherapy & Essential Oils for Healing Common Ailments, Beauty, Stress & Anxiety) + CARRIER OILS FOR BEGINNERS (Discover the Characteristics & Beauty & Health Benefits of Carrier Oils for Mixing Aromatherapy Essential Oils) + ESSENTIAL OILS & AROMATHERAPY FOR BEGINNERS (Secrets to Beauty & weight Loss Using Proven Essential Oil & Aromatherapy Recipes) + NATURAL HOMEMADE CLEANING RECIPES FOR BEGINNERS (Essential Oil Recipes for Household Cleaning, Laundry & Toxic Free Living)

http://www.amazon.com/BOX-SET-12-Essential-Aromatherapy-ebook/dp/B00KCBCHE4

BOX SET #13: SUPERFOODS THAT KICKSTART YOUR WEIGHT LOSS (Learn How to Use 30 Superfoods to Boost Weight Loss, Immunity and to Live a Healthier Lifestyle) + ESSENTIAL OILS & AROMATHERAPY FOR BEGINNERS (Secrets to Beauty, Health and Weight Loss Using Proven Essential Oil and Aromatherapy Recipes) + BODY BUTTERS FOR BEGINNERS (Proven Secrets To Making All Natural Body Butters For Rejuvenating And Hydrating Your Skin) + SOAP MAKING FOR BEGINNERS (A Guide to Making Natural Homemade Soaps from Scratch, Includes Recipes and Step by Step Processes for Making Soaps) + HOMEMADE BODY SCRUBS FOR BEGINNERS (50 Proven All Natural, Easy Recipes For Body Scrub & Facial Masks To Exfoliate, Nourish, & Care For Your Skin)

http://www.amazon.com/BOX-SET-Superfoods-Kickstart-Aromatherapy-ebook/dp/B00KC8G6DK/

BOX SET 14: Essential Oils & Weight Loss for Beginners (Ultimate Guide to Losing Weight, Increasing Energy, Balancing Metabolism & Appetite Using Essential Oils & Aromatherapy) + Apple Cider Vinegar for Beginners (Proven

Secrets Using Apple Cider Vinegar for Health, Weight Loss, and Skin Care) + Body Butters For Beginners (Proven Secrets To Making All Natural Body Butters For Rejuvenating And Hydrating Your Skin)
+ Homemade Body Scrubs & Masks for Beginners (50 Proven All Natural, Easy Recipes for Body Scrub & Facial Masks to Exfoliate, Nourish, & Care for Your Skin) + Coconut Oil for Easy Weight Loss (A Step by Step Guide for Using Virgin Coconut Oil for Quick and Easy Weight Loss)

http://www.amazon.com/BOX-SET-Essential-Beginners-Aromatherapy-ebook/dp/B00KEDO68U

If the links do not work, for whatever reason, you can simply search for these titles on the Amazon website to find them.

Superfoods that Kickstart Your Weight Loss Learn How to Use 30 Superfoods to Boost Weight Loss, Immunity and to Live a Healthier Lifestyle

Made in the USA
San Bernardino, CA
18 April 2018